Cure Tooth Decay

How to Prevent & Cure Tooth Decay & Cavities Naturally in the Comfort of Your Own Home

By Fiona Hathaway

Table of Contents

Copyright

or directions contained within is the solitary and utter responsibility of the recipient reader.

Under no circumstances will any legal responsibility or blame be held against the publisher for any reparation, damages, or monetary loss due to the information herein, either directly or indirectly.

Respective authors own all copyrights not held by the publisher.

The information herein is offered for informational purposes solely, and is universal as so. The presentation of the information is without contract or any type of guarantee assurance.

The trademarks that are used are without any consent, and the publication of the trademark is without permission or backing by the trademark owner. All trademarks and brands within this book are for clarifying purposes only and are the owned by the owners themselves, not affiliated with this document.

Introduction

Confidence, there is no better way of showing confidence than by standing upright with good posture and having a white, toothy grin plastered upon the face. It is a combination of both mental conditioning and pride in the physical form. However, it is hard to smile when the teeth are infested with cavities.

Around 90% of the overall population has dental cavities, and the statistics only worsen with age. It has been found that 28% of children 5 years old and below have cavities and that a greater portion (about 87%) of the adult population, namely those aged 20 to 39, suffer from this. However, saying that tooth decay comes with aging is erroneous. Poor nutrition and lack of the essential vitamins and minerals that contribute to dental health are among the major reasons behind the drastic increase in figures of tooth decay cases. The condition of the teeth gives away many secrets of an individual's lifestyle and it is therefore important to take care of them.

This eBook will address such concerns by discussing the anatomy of the tooth, followed by a detailed explanation of the causes of cavities. This is imperative in determining how one should deal with these carries. Also, this eBook will talk about proper tooth care and some affordable and effective home remedies for cavities.

Read on and discover some surprising facts about the teeth.

Chapter 1: The Anatomy of the Tooth

The teeth are some of the hardest substances in the body. They are mainly used for mastication and they also aid in speech. The average human adult should have 32 permanent teeth in total, with 28 of these erupting at 13 years old and the last 4 (the wisdom teeth) appearing at 18 years of age.

pThe Layers of a Tooth

The tooth has three distinct layers, namely the enamel, dentin and pulp. Cavities always affect the outermost layer first and slowly dig their way to the inner portion. The more layers that are affected, the greater the damage dealt by the decay.

Enamel

This is the outermost part of the tooth, which serves as a protection for the inner structures. It is made mostly out of a rock hard mineral called Calcium Phosphatase, which contributes to its sturdiness.

Dentin

After the enamel comes the dentin. It produces a tough mineral substance and contains numerous tubes that connect to the pulp.

Pulp

This is located at the center of the tooth. This is softer compared to the other 2 layers and serves as the living quarters of nerves and blood vessels. Damage to this area will cause pain.

The Parts of the Tooth

The tooth, though small, is made up of several parts. Each of which has a distinct function.

Crown

In terms of structure, the crown is the topmost and most visible part of the tooth. The form or shape of this part determines the function of the tooth.

Cementum

This is a connective tissue that fastens the roots of the teeth to the gums and, subsequently, to the jawbone, preventing it from falling off.

Periodontal Ligament

This is a tissue that, like the cementum, aids in keeping the teeth attached to the gums and jawbone.

Gumline

This is the area where the gums and teeth meet. There is a small groove formed at this area so, without proper brushing technique, plaque or tartar may accumulate and result to various gum and tooth disorders.

Root

This is the bottommost part of the tooth, which comprises about 2/3 of the entire structure. It is implanted into the jawbone.

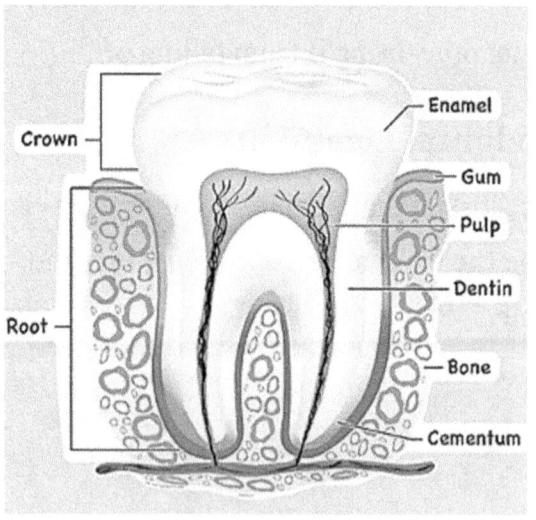

Different Kinds of Teeth

All humans have a predetermined arrangement and number of teeth regarding its external structure. There are 5 types in total: incisors, canines, molars, premolars, and wisdom teeth.

Incisors

These are located at the front most part of the jaw and are shaped like a chisel. There are 8 in total, with 4 at the top and 4 at the bottom. As the name suggests, these function to cut food.

Canines

Also known as cuspids, these teeth have pointed crowns and serve as the boundary between the premolars and the incisors. There are 4 in total. Because they are sharp, they are used to tear the food the incisors cannot.

Premolars

Premolars are also known as bicuspids because they have two pointed tips (cusps) at the crown. These grow in between the canines and the molars and are mainly used to crush and/or tear food.

Molars

The crowns of these teeth are flat and are used in grinding or chewing food. There are three of these that are lined up at each side of the jaw (upper left, upper right, lower left, lower right), which equates to a total of 12.

3rd Molars a.k.a. Wisdom Teeth

These teeth are the last to erupt, often appearing by the time one turns 18 years old. In most cases, the wisdom teeth have to be taken out as they tend to congest the area where they grow and may impede the growth of the surrounding structures.

Non-Congenital Dental Disorders

Poor dental hygiene and inattention to malformations of the structures of the oral cavity could lead to a variety of conditions.

Dental Carries

More commonly known as cavities, these are formed when bacteria accumulate at the enamel. It evades the area and, if not addressed, will dig through the layers of the tooth and may affect adjacent teeth. These are mostly found on the molars and premolars.

Tooth Decay

Most people would erroneously interchange 'tooth decay' with or use it synonymously with 'cavities.' However, unbeknownst to most, tooth decay is a general term which encompasses all diseases of the teeth – a category where cavities fall under. If left untreated, it may lead to more serious conditions such as infection, pain and loss of the affected tooth.

Plaque

This is a thick, sticky, colorless substance formed by clumped up bacteria and their secretions. Sugar-rich foods are the main culprit for the formation of this substance. However, one can easily remove it by brushing the teeth.

Tartar

Failure to remove plaque allows the substance to merge with the surrounding minerals and form a harder substance called tartar. Unlike plaque, removing this is not possible by brushing alone. It needs professional intervention (a.k.a. a visit to the dentist).

Periodontis

'-Itis' is a suffix which refers to inflammation.

This means that periodontis is the inflammation of the periodontal cavity (which includes the deeper structures of the mouth).

Gingivitis

This is the inflammation of the gums, usually starting at the gum line. This is usually caused by the buildup of plaque and tartar at the gums.

Tooth Sensitivity

Teeth are normally durable and are capable of handling hot or cold temperatures. However, once the dentin is exposed, the teeth become sensitive to the temperatures they were once able to withstand. This is called tooth sensitivity.

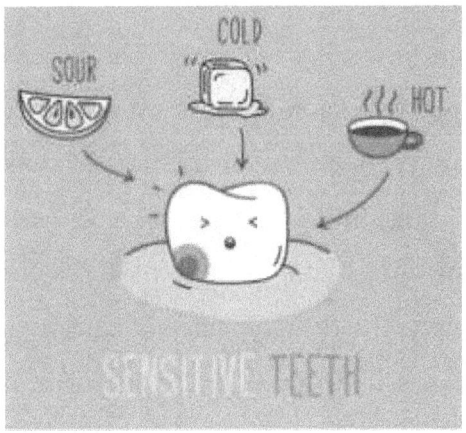

Chapter 2: Why We Get Cavities

The main culprit for tooth decay is bacteria, which comes in the form of plaque. This substance lives off of glucose and secretes acidic substances that corrode the teeth. Additionally, the hypothalamus and parotid glands that control the flow of fluid in the minuscule channels in the teeth, affect the growth of cavities. Now, the big question is what are the factors that increase one's susceptibility to tooth decay?

Millions of years ago, there were no dentists, dental care products, or the like. However, Dr. Melvin Page and Dr. Weston Price, two highly acclaimed dentists, have pointed out the lack of, or even the total absence of cavities in early human fossils from all over the world. As a matter of fact, their teeth should've experienced greater wear and tear due to their diet, which mainly consists of tough protein and at times, raw vegetables and fruits. This is sheer proof that teeth were built to last a lifetime. Then why do so many people (90% of the population, to be exact) suffer from tooth decay? Perhaps, it is the very diet of the early humans that has strengthened their teeth.

Modern man's diet consists mainly of starches, which are rich in glucose and a lot of processed foods jam packed with preservatives and Phytic Acid. Eating these creates a breeding ground for bacteria in the mouth. Furthermore, teeth weaken when there is an imbalance of the levels of essential minerals (phosphorus, magnesium and calcium) and fat-soluble vitamins (D, K, E and A) in the blood.

However, although the diet is a major contributor to dental health, other factors may also influence the occurrence of tooth decay:

Dental Hygiene

Poor dental hygiene or brushing technique is a definite cause of cavities, so is the inability to remove food that is stuck in between the teeth. Not visiting the dentist regularly and having teeth cleaned impedes accurate assessment of dental health.

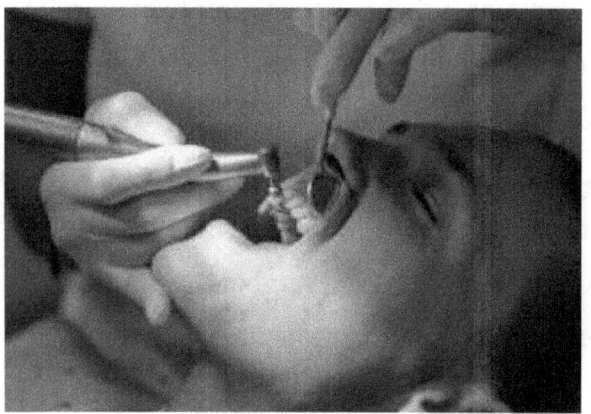

Medical Conditions

Diabetes involves an inability of the body to regulate glucose levels. As aforementioned, glucose serves as food for bacteria and high amounts of this will increase the amount of plaque in the mouth. Also, eating disorders such as bulimia and anorexia nervosa involve the constant act of purging, which expels the acidic contents of the stomach from the body. These pass through the internal structures of the oral cavity – including the teeth. Doing so repetitively will thin out the enamel, thus causing damage to the teeth.

Additionally, since these people often suffer from dehydration, there is a deficiency on the production of saliva, which is an important element that regulates pH levels in the mouth. GERD (gastroesophageal reflux disease), which is also known as heartburn, works in a similar way to vomiting. The main difference is that only a little amount of stomach acid is refluxed into the mouth. This can still dissolve the enamel of the teeth and is also a point of concern.

Other Factors

Teething children are more vulnerable to bacterial invasion of the tooth because newly erupted teeth are initially weaker and more susceptible to damage from acid. Also, the location of the tooth influences the occurrence of tooth decay. It often affects molars and premolars (teeth at the back of the mouth) as these contain multiple grooves where food particles can accumulate.

Having a dry mouth (usually due to too little saliva) also increases the risk of acquiring cavities as saliva neutralizes pH in the mouth, washes off most sugars and food particles. This may be caused by a variety of health conditions such as xerostomia, Sjögren's syndrome, mouth breathing, aging or dehydration. Moreover, fluoride deficiency is another point of concern as fluoride protects teeth from acid produced by bacteria.

Symptoms of Tooth Decay

The initial stages of decay usually bear no obvert symptoms. These only arise when an infection or a cavity has developed. The most common of which is toothache. This is usually followed by inflammation of the gums surrounding the affected tooth, halitosis and/or a bad taste in the mouth, and tooth discoloration (e.g. brown, gray, or black spots).

Diagnosis

When any of the aforementioned symptoms occur, do see a dentist to have the problem addressed and the condition diagnosed. Upon visit, the dentist will first ask a series of questions in order for him or her to gain an accurate account of the client's dental history. Some questions include prior dental problems and routine tooth care.

Then, the dentist shall assess the condition of the teeth with the use of a small mirror and a pointed tool. In some cases, the dentist will let the client have an x-ray of the teeth to visualize the presence of tooth decay more accurately.

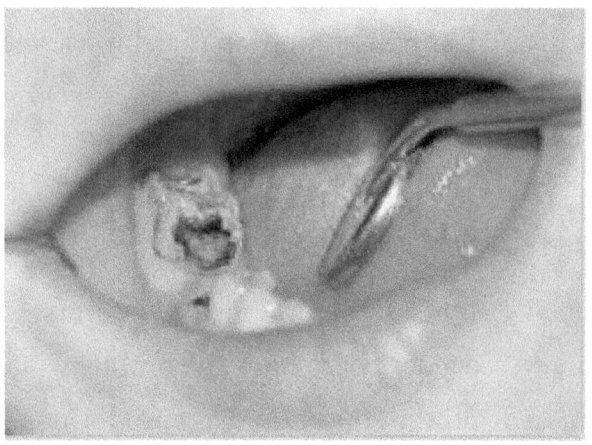

Chapter 3: Taking Care of Those Pearly Whites

Prevention is better than cure. Ensuring that the teeth are clean, healthy, and properly maintained does not only serve aesthetic purposes, but is also integral in communication, normal development of the surrounding structures (such as the gums and jaw), and can also raise one's self esteem.   Once teeth have been damaged, they can never return to their previous state and they become more fragile. Hygiene requirements also become more demanding.

Taking care of the teeth is imperative as it prevents diseases of the gums and teeth that subsequently allow one to save money from potential reparative visits to the dentist. There is a decreased need for fillings or other additional procedures, which makes the bi-yearly dental checkup more pleasant while allowing one to spend much less time on the dentist's chair.

Tooth decay is unpleasant and often painful. Prevention of such will allow the teeth to last long and decrease the need for dentures upon reaching old age. It also improves overall health and one's hygiene (prevents halitosis). Also, it keeps the teeth nice and pearly white, which allows one to have a beautiful smile.

Basic dental hygiene involves three integral practices: daily flossing and brushing of the teeth, proper nutrition, and bi-yearly visits to the dentist.

Brushing the Teeth

Teeth should be brushed at least twice a day — once after eating the first meal of the day and once before hitting the hay as it removes plaque.

Make sure that each session lasts for a minimum of 2 minutes and that all surfaces have been cleaned.

Don't brush right after eating, especially after a highly acidic meal (carbonated beverages, fruit, wine, etc.) as it may do more harm than good. Wait for at least 1 hour after a meal to allow the saliva to interact with the acid in the mouth and neutralize its pH. Also, avoid eating or drinking anything approximately 30 minutes after the teeth have been brushed at it washes out the protective action of the toothpaste.

Proper Technique

The brush must be at about a 45° angle from the gum line. Brush the teeth with gentle, circular strokes. Be sure to brush every tooth and every portion, including the inside and outside areas. Afterwards, clean the tongue with a tongue scraper.

Refrain from rinsing the oral cavity with water or mouthwash after brushing as it washes away the protective qualities of the toothpaste. Instead, spit out the excess toothpaste into the sink.

Children 7 years old and below should be supervised when brushing the teeth. Make sure that they only apply a pea sized amount and that they do not swallow the toothpaste.

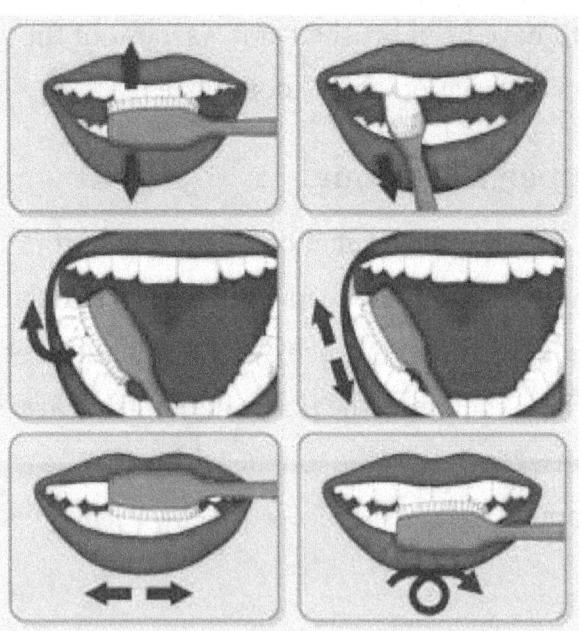

Looking for the Right Toothbrush

Both the electric and manual toothbrush are equally good, it is just a matter of personal preference. In choosing a manual toothbrush, look for compact, round-ended, medium or soft bristles (hard bristles are harmful). Make sure that it has a small head and there is a mixture of long and short bristle strands. For an electrical toothbrush, it is recommended to choose one with an oscillating or rotating head.

Interdental brushes are special brushes with a single tuft that can be used as an alternative for dental floss. It is effective in cleaning hard-to-reach areas. Consult the dentist for the proper type to suit individual needs.

The toothbrush should be replaced every 2-3 months as they experience wear and tear with each use – it makes them less effective in cleaning the teeth.

Looking for the Right Toothpaste

The toothpaste should be approved by American Dental Association and should contain fluoride as it prevents tooth decay. Children 7 years old and above (including adults) should use family toothpaste, which contains 1,350-1,500 ppm of fluoride. Children 6 years old and below should use toothpaste with at least 1,000 ppm.

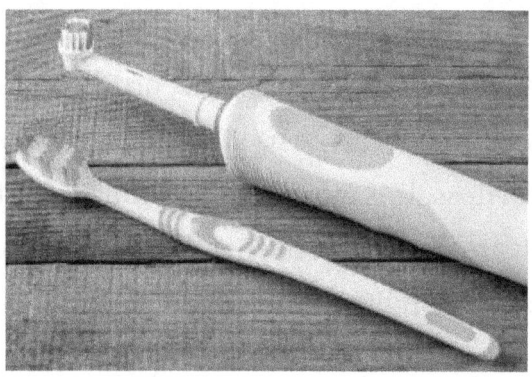

Flossing

Flossing involves the use of a thin, sturdy string like object that is about 12-18 inches long.

To use, grasp each end and insert it in the spaces between the teeth. Move with 8 – 10 back-and-forth strokes to remove the unwanted particles. It is effective in removing food particles and plaque.

Since dental floss can fit into hard-to-reach areas such as the spaces in between the teeth, it should be used in adjunct with tooth brushing as the toothbrush cannot reach these areas.

Do not use toothpicks as these can damage the gums.

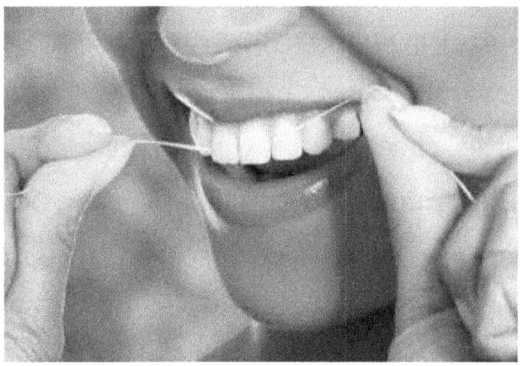

Gargling Mouthwash

Mouthwash contains antibacterial properties that can kill off the harmful bacteria in the mouth, prevents gum disease, and washes out plaque. Ideally, it should contain fluoride and must be alcohol-free. Do not use this right after
brushing the teeth as it can damage them. Instead, use at separate occasions, such as after meals. After gargling, do not consume anything within 30 minutes.

Eating Right

The following foods are good for the teeth: fruits, vegetables, whole grains (freshly prepared), dairy products (such as yellow butter, cheese and raw milk), unsweetened coffee, internal organs such as liver, bone marrow or bone broths, sea foods. High fiber foods stimulate saliva production and drinking tea, specifically black and green tea, as well as cranberry juice can diminish the growth of bacteria and the formation of plaque.

Stay well hydrated. Drinking water does not only wash out bacteria, but it also is a key factor in the production of saliva. It is also good for one to chew sugar-free gum after meals. It also stimulates saliva production, which is capable of decreasing acidity in the mouth; too much of which can damage the teeth.

Be sure to have a diet rich in important vitamins (A, D, E, K) and essential minerals (calcium, magnesium, phosphorus, etc.).

Lifestyle Choices

Visit the dentist once every 6 months to have the teeth cleaned. Do not smoke as tobacco and tobacco products do not only cause debilitating health problems, but can also damage the dental enamel and cause oral cancer.

Pediatric Considerations

Before a child turns 1 year old, or about 6 months after the child starts teething (whichever comes first), he or she should be brought to the dentist to have the teeth assessed for potential dental problems.

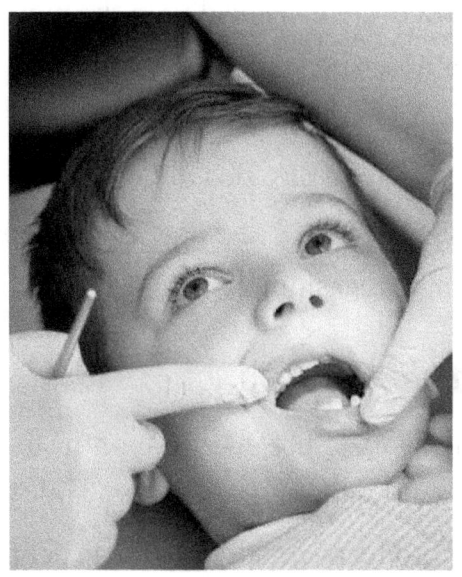

Chapter 4: Dealing with Tooth Decay

Once damage affects the teeth, it cannot be fully undone. Despite the various treatment modalities employed to heal the damaged teeth, the traces of damage cannot fully disappear. The teeth have reached a more vulnerable state and therefore need extra attention and care.

Medical Treatment

Medical intervention depends on the severity of the tooth decay. During the early stages, prior to the formation of a cavity, intervention is a simple as brushing the teeth with fluoride-rich products. However, once the bacteria dug through the enamel, the dentist may recommend one or a combination of the following:

Filling - this is the removal of the decayed portion and subsequent filling up of the hole with a special material.

Crown or cap - this is the installation of an artificial crown to replace severe, badly damaged portions of the teeth.

Root canal - it is the recommended for infected pulp. It involves the removal of the diseased portion.

Extraction - this is the removal of the entire tooth, which will then be replaced with any of the following: bridge or implant. It is recommended when there is severe, irreparable damage on the tooth.

For pain and inflammation, place ice packs onto the cheek near affected teeth or gums. Keep this on for about 10 to 15 minutes and perform constantly throughout the day.

Be sure to place a dry cloth in between the cold pack and the cheek to protect the skin from extreme cold.

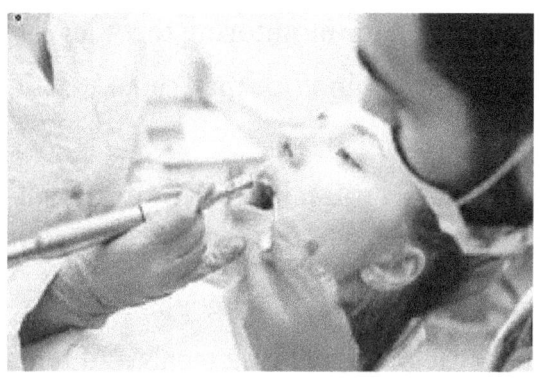

Tooth Remineralization

In order to be adequately nourished, one must
eat the way the human body was designed to
eat. To do so, three main changes must be
made to the diet:

Avoid consuming processed grains, bagels,
breakfast cereals, sodas, and other processed
foodstuff as they can cause ebb and flow of
blood sugar levels.

Through the course of time, the glands responsible for monitoring these levels become tired and this may cause cavities.

Monitor sugar intake. Avoid sugar-rich foods (bacteria thrive in glucose-rich environments). If unavoidable, only eat sugar-rich foods during meals and not for snacks or alone without anything else. Natural sugars are the preferred choices, but still, consume these in moderation. Unbeknownst to most, some fruits have been genetically modified to be sweeter and bigger to meet mass production needs. Blueberries, dates, and bananas in particular contain high levels of sugar. Stevia and raw honey are healthier alternatives.

Increase consumption of Activator X – a vital component in teeth mineralization.
It is found in dairy products derived from the milk of grass-eating cattle.

It contains a fertility factor that sends signals to the hormonal systems of the body which, in turn, stimulate the production and growth of healthy teeth and bones. Numerous studies have found that the growth of cavities in subjects who consumed these high quality dairy products was impeded and, ultimately, halted. In fact, some have reported the growth of new teeth structures and whiter, healthier teeth. It is recommended to consume 1 tbsp. of this butter or at least 1 glass of raw milk per day.

Decreasing Phytic Acid in the Diet

Phytic Acid is an antioxidant compound that is found abundantly in seeds, grains, beans and nuts. The problem with this substance is that it binds on to enzymes and minerals in the body (calcium, zinc, manganese and iron), which decreases the speed of their absorption.

Furthermore, they also leech off the minerals found in the teeth and other bodily structures. Due to this parasitic action, the body experiences digestive problems, lacks nutrition, there is a lack of appetite, and there is formation of tooth decay.

Ancient methods of food preparation which kill off about 50-100% of the phytic acid present in food, particularly sourdough fermentation and sprouting, have been discontinued. This is why the effects of this substance are more apparent today than they were before.

As a solution, simply limit the intake of grains and avoid unfermented soy products.

Also, since there are higher levels of Phytol in foods fertilized with high-phosphate materials, it is advisable to look for organic, GMO-free foods.

Home Made Mineralized Toothpaste

Buying toothpaste that has been reinforced with fluoride is a bit more costly than purchasing the regular kind. Also, since these are commercialized products, there isn't an adequate amount of fluoride incorporated into the mix. To create a homemade solution that is cheaper yet perhaps even more effective than these branded tubes, simply mix I the following ingredients: 20 drops of an essential oil (either peppermint or clove), 4 tbsp. coconut oil, 20 drops trace minerals (either magnesium or calcium powder), 1 tbsp. xylitol (an alternative to this would be 1/8 tsp. stevia), and 2 tbsp. aluminum-free baking soda.

Oil Pulling

This is an ancient method that has been used for hundreds of years that is capable of detoxifying the oral cavity and, subsequently, killing off the substances that cause tooth decay. As a matter of fact, it has also been found to alleviate headaches and cure some systematic ailments such as diabetes. This simple method requires one to gargle a tablespoon of oil (sunflower, sesame, coconut or MCT) for about 20 minutes. Afterwards, spit the oil out and quickly rinse it off with warm water or with a salt water solution to provide additional antibacterial benefits. One can then resume with regular dental care and brush the teeth.

Oil pulling should be done every day upon waking up. It is important to note that the oil spit out may appear yellowish or milky white. This is normal and should not be a cause of worry.

Herbs, Spices and Other Household Ingredients

Some household items can aid in the alleviation of the symptoms that come with tooth decay and even cure the said condition.

Salt

Salt has long been known as a powerful antibacterial, which allows it to halt the growth of bacteria and plaque, and an antiseptic, which prevents infection of wounded structures. It is also effective in easing up pain.

Dissolve 1 tsp. of salt in a glass of lukewarm water and swish the solution in the mouth for an entire minute to achieve the desired effect. Ensure that the solution passes through the affected area. Repeat this process 3 times a day, every day until tooth ache is alleviated.

One may also blend half a teaspoon of salt with mustard oil or lemon extract to create a paste-like consistency. Massage this onto the gums for a couple of minutes to kill of harmful bacteria, then immediately gargle lukewarm water afterwards. Do this twice a day, every day.

Indian Gooseberry

Also, known as amla, this is an antioxidant-rich herb that can disinfect the mouth and therefore prevent infection.   Moreover, since it is also rich in ascorbic acid, it is capable of promoting connective tissue growth, as well as boosting the healing process.

One could eat this herb on a daily basis. Alternatively, one could also mix ½ tsp. of dried Indian Gooseberry powder in half a glass of water and drink it daily.

Nutmeg

This delicious spice has been found by a group of researchers from Yonsei University, Korea to have anticarcinogenic properties, which can be used to prevent the appearance of tooth decay caused by carcinogenic substances in the mouth.

To use, simply mix a bit of clove oil with some grated nutmeg and apply it onto the damaged teeth. Allow it to stay for about 10 minutes prior to rinsing the mouth with lukewarm drinking water. This should be done 3-4 times in a 24-hour period.

Garlic

This contains rich antibacterial properties that aid in the alleviation of the symptoms of tooth decay. It is also a potent antiseptic, which promotes teeth and gum health.

Crush about 3-4 cloves of garlic and mix it with a quarter of a teaspoon of salt to create a paste. Gently dab this onto the affected teeth and allow it to stay for about 10 minutes. Afterwards, rinse it off with mouthwash. Perform this procedure twice a day, every day until symptoms subside.

Alternatively, rubbing garlic oil or chewing on a raw clove of garlic could produce similar results.

Clove

This plant is a potent pain reliever that possesses anti-inflammatory properties that can reduce pain and swelling caused by dental carries. Additionally, it is also an antibacterial that serves to inhibit the growth of plaque and prevent further spread of the carries. Use this in moderation as it only provides temporary relief.

There are two ways to utilize this plant.

The first method is to dilute 2-3 drops of its oil extract in ¼ tsp. of sesame seed oil.

Then, use a cotton ball to absorb the solution and gently dab it onto the affected area. This should be done at least once a day, every day before going to bed.

The second method is chewing the raw clove whole until its oils are extracted. Then, let it stay underneath the tongue for a couple of minutes.

Conclusion

Thank you for purchasing this book "Cure Tooth Decay: How to Prevent & Cure Tooth Decay & Cavities Naturally in the Comfort of Your Own Home."

Hopefully, it was able to successfully teach the basics of tooth decay – its causes, symptoms and the required treatments. Furthermore, the author hopes that the aforementioned home remedies and interventions proved to be both convenient and effective in dealing with dental problems.

Continue practicing good dental habits until they become a part of the routine. Remember, healthy teeth and gums are the mark of a clean and physically healthy individual.

www.ingramcontent.com/pod-product-compliance
Lightning Source LLC
Chambersburg PA
CBHW071007180526
45168CB00003B/1326